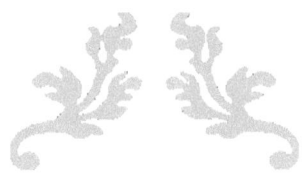

THOU SHALT EAT

A Guide to Nutrition That Even Doctors Can Understand

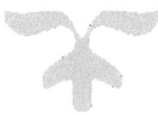

LULU PRESS

Thou Shalt Eat

Dedication

This book is dedicated to Donald "Donnie" Young, my brother who died at the tender age of five. WE ARE BECAUSE YOU WERE. I am grateful that God has granted me the skills and abilities to be able to achieve my current successes, pursue my future and author this book.

Jer. 29:11 – "For I know the plans that I have for you"

Foreword

Preface

I am glad you have decided to learn more about health, wellness and of course nutrition.

For many of us, these are often areas of great interest, but also areas of great informational deficiencies. Food is however, an essential part to life, a basic human need. It surprised me, that everyone eats food, must of us enjoy food, but no one ever seems to truly understand food. I decided to finally write this book, when talking with my godmother about health disparities and nutritional issues with our family. She begged me to share more information with her on how to live a healthier life. It shocked me how enthused she was. I began to wonder, how many people actually want to know about nutrition. It is something that a majority of people desire? Do people care about their health? The more I pondered these questions, the more I realized the answer was yes. In addition, to those who didn't want to learn about nutrition, they just didn't know that they wanted to learn about it. They complained of their weight, their energy, their health and their risk factors. So, I couldn't resist the urge to share the knowledge that I have acquired with those who don't know. I also wanted this book to be an easy read for anyone. I wanted teens and adults alike to understand, whether or not they have a medical degree or are a health professional. I wanted literacy to be the only hindrance in someone not gaining access to this information, that when applied can be life saving. That is also why this text is slightly larger. I didn't want poor eyesight or an eternity of squinting to be the cause of someone not getting this information about food.

Twelve Commandments

Thou Shalt Eat

Getting Started:

How I Became Interested in Nutrition

"The importance of a goal should not first be in setting a date to accomplish that goal, but the first step should be determining when you are truly ready to begin"

-Getting Started-

I remember stepping onto my college campus on the first day of orientation week filled with excitement and anticipation. I was eleven hours away from home, and finally on my own. It was at this moment, that for the first time I was making all of the decisions. I choose when I would wake up, when I would go to sleep, what time I set the curfew, who I choose my friends, and what I was going to eat. I had the independence to choose my food. But with that freedom came responsibility. I had the freedom to choose whatever I ate, that meant I had the power to make decisions about my health.

For many of us, this power is limited. Whether it is money, resources, availability, transportation, storage or a range of many other limiting factors, for the most part, we still have this power of choice. The question then becomes whether or not we choose to exercise that power in a way that is physiologically responsible to our bodies.

So as I began to exercise the right to choose whatever foods I wanted to consume, I began to feel empowered to eat as much pizza, burgers, creamy and cheesy pasta, buffets of desserts and generous amounts of salt, washed down with sweetened teas. I continued this trend more months after I entered college. This combined with limited sleep and stress lead me to what most would consider very poor health. Some days I could not remember the last time I had eaten something green (vegetables). The problem with this habitual unhealthy lifestyle was that I could not see what it was doing to my body internally.

What changed for me was one class that I took in college in Food Studies. I never intended to major in food or nutrition, or to even take a single course in that field; I was a committed business major. Nevertheless, during my freshman year, I needed an extra course outside of my business classes, and since I loved to eat food, I decided to take Food Studies I.

That course changed my life. The professor was a former dietician who had worked in healthcare, culinary, private practice, federal, non-profit and in the corporate sector. But what set her apart in my mind was that she had earned her degree in agriculture, which meant she understood how food was produced, and that food was a business (which was very important to a business major). Throughout the course, I learned that food is not just a common indulgence, but is an interdisciplinary system that affects everyone. One particular aspect of food stuck with me, that aspect was nutrition.

As I began to learn more about nutrition, I started to see that I needed to make changes in my personal diet. But that was not enough. I knew that other people, people that I knew, my family, friends and colleagues, also could use this information. After this realization, I changed my major to Food Studies and Nutrition.

I.

Book of Nutrition:

A Brief Description of Nutrition

"Nutrition is what you eat, who you get it from, how much you eat it, when you eat it and what happens after you eat it. Nutrition is everything that you wish you didn't have to worry about when you sit down to eat"

-Nutrition-

In the United States of America, nutrition has definitely been all but forgotten. It seems that people do not truly care about their bodies, or understand how to care for them. People also seem to forget the fact that food, the physical matter that we eat, is what affects our nutrition.

For example, water is a vital part of a healthy diet, but annually the average American will only consume twenty-five gallons of water, compared to thirty gallons of milk, and compared to fifty gallons of soda. That means that Americans drink double the amount of soda as they do water. Even though water is an essential part of good nutrition. This is partly because there is such a big business in food.

There are thirty-three billion dollars spent every year on food advertising; ten billion dollars are spent just on advertisements specific to children. Many cultural aspects of food affect the industry and nutrition as a whole. The world now desires convenience; microwavable foods, premade, prepackaged, frozen, quick preparation and instant meals. Along with this change comes economic shifts; if the consumer wants it, the consumer gets it.

As important as nutrition is in our quality of life, it has been reduced to label checking for fat, salt and calories. Nutrition is a broad topical science, a large body of food related knowledge; it is the science of food and its components that work together in the body to promote good health and well-being. Nutrition is not an opinion; it is a factual, proven and reliable science. Nutrients are the chemical substances in food that contribute to health and an essential diet nutrients. They provide calories to give us energy and regulate the processes of the body. Nutrients provide energy, growth, development and maintenance to the body.

Food studies notes

- We need a diet with fruit, vegetables and grains, along with plenty of exercise

- 70,000 meals, 120,000 pounds of food, 3 to 4 years eating

- Flavor texture and appearance are the most important factors in determining food choices

- Early influences, routines and habits affect food choices

o 100 basic items is 75% of all food intake

☐ Most Americans eat

- 30 gallons of milk on avg

- 25 gallons of bottled water

- 50 gallons of soda

- Americans drink double the amount of soda as water or milk

- 33 billion is spent on food advertising

- 10 billion is specific to children

- Social changes
  o Convenience
    □ Microwave
    □ Premade
    □ Frozen
    □ Quick prep
  o Economics
    □ 12% of income spent on food
  o Nutrition
    □ What we consider healthy
    □ Label checking
- For calories
- For fat
- For salt
- For vitamins
- Hunger – drive to find food and eat
- Appetite- influences that encourage us to find food and eat food often when hungry
- Satiety- no desire to eat, satisfaction
- Nutrients- chemical substances in food that contribute to health, and an essential diet nutrients, they provide calories to give us energy needs to regulate the processes of the body

- Essential nutrients- substance that when left out of diet, result in poor health, the body cant produce this nutrient or cant produce enough to meet the needs of the body, if added back to the diet before permeant damage then the affected aspects of health are restored

- Carb- compound containing, carbon, hydrogen, and oxygen, sugars starches and fiber

- Lipid- highly carbon and hydrogen little oxygen compounds don't dissolve in water

- Protein- food and body compounds made of amino acids

- Vitamin- compounds that regulate and support chemical reactions

- Mineral- element that promotes chemical reactions to form body structures

- Water-universal solvent, body is 60%, H2O, 9 cups a day for women, 13 cups a day for men

- Kilocalorie- heat energy

- Simple sugar- mon or disaccharides

- Complex carbs- composed of many mono and di's like starch and fiber

- Macronutrient- nutrient needed in gram quantities

- Micronutrients- nutrient needed in milligram quantities

- Cell- basis of life organization that contain genetic material and synthesize material

- Bond- link between two atoms

- Fiber- substances in plant food not digested by the processes that take place in the stomach and intestine, adding bulk to feces. Fiber found naturally in food is called dietary fiber

- Enzyme- speeds the rate of chemical reactions but not altered by reaction

- Amino acid- the building block for all proteins containing carbon and nitrogen

- chemical reaction- interaction between two chemicals

- inorganic- lacking carbon bonded to hydrogen

- electrolytes- substances that break down into ions in water and are able to conduct an electric current

- solvent-a liquid in which other substances dissolve

- metabolism- chemical processes in the body by which energy is provided in useful forms and vital activities are sustained.

- phytochemical- plant chemical that can reduce cancer and heart disease risks

- salt- compound of sodium and chloride in a 40:60 ratio

- compound- types of atoms bonded together in definite proportion

- alcohol- ethyl or ethanol

- genes- specific segments of chromosomes that are blueprints to all body proteins

- diet- food and beverages that is consumed

- Nutrition is broad topical science, a large body of food related knowledge

  o Nutrition- is the science of food and its components that work together in the body to promote good health and well being

  ☐ It is not an opinion, it is a factual, proven, and reliable science

- Importance

  o By 6 years old the brain of a child has been vastly influenced by their food

  o Food is a basic need

- Food insecurity- not knowing when, what, or in what quantity or quality of food , one will consume

- Essential nutrients- nutrients that are found in food but not produced by the body

- Nutrients

  o Provide energy, growth, development and maintenance

  o Regulate the bodies functions

- ☐ Metabolic functions- Water vitamins minerals
- ☐ Development and growth- protein
- ☐ Energy- carbs and fat
- Food- gives nutrients and non- nutrients

- Energy
- o Carbohydrates (CHO's) and Lipids (fats)
- ☐ Energy output measured in calories
- ☐ 1 gram of CHO= 4 cal.
- ☐ 1 gram of fat= 9 cal.
- ☐ 1 tsp= 1 gram
- ☐ 3 tbsp.= 1 tsp
- Growth and Development
- o Protein
- Metabolic Functions
- o Such as
- ☐ Digestion
- ☐ Excretion
- ☐ Heart rate
- ☐ Cardiovascular functions

- ☐ Lung Activity

- ☐ Energy Conversion

- o Vitamins, Minerals, and water

- • Six Categories of nutrients

- o Water

- o Minerals

- o Vitamins

- o CHO

- ☐ Sugar is a carbohydrate

- o Fat

- o Protein

- ☐ Are broken down to 40 to 50+

- ☐ Listed on DOC 3

- • Non- Nutrients

- o Phyto= plant

- o Phytochemical, phytonutrient, antioxidant

- o Antioxidant

- ☐ Chemical substance that prevents peroxidation and free radicals

- ☐ Peroxidation: destruction of cells, food, organs, and cell reproductive structures by producing free radicals that aid aging, spoilage, promote cancer formation and diseases

- ☐ Some vitamins are antioxidants

- A= beta carotene
- C= ascorbic acid
- E
  o Phytonutrients
    □ Mainly plant bases
      - Vegetables
      - Fruits
      - Grains
      - Nuts
      - Seeds
      - Spices
      - Herbs
      - Oils
- Risks of Not Eating Nutrients and Non Nutrients Properly
  o Too much bad CHO= heart disease
  o Too many sodium based minerals= stroke, high blood pressure
- Colors of health
  o Orange= beta carotene
  o Dark Green= chlorophyll
  o Bright Green= chlorophyll and beta carotene
- Aroma

o　　　Smells of food comes from its nutrients

•　　　Rancidity: the destruction to the lipids and cell membranes and changes the normal function of the fat causing spoilage or the normal function of the cell causing cell mutation and cell death

•　　　Article

o　　　The science of nutrition

☐　　　Source

•　　　Sizer and Whitney 12th edition

•　　　Pp 13-15

☐　　　Science

•　　　Research to get a process

•　　　Hypothesis and theory

•　　　Methodology to obtain accurate data

☐　　　Nutrition is a field of knowledge, formed of organized facts

☐　　　It is a young science

☐　　　"Most nutrition research started before 1900" BUT

☐　　　Early chemistry found many nutritional facts as early as 1700, but it wasn't considered nutrition

☐　　　Nutrition science is an active and changing science and is often contradictory

☐　　　Many facts in nutrition are known with certainty with the backing of other sciences

- ☐ Reading is a part of research
- ☐
- • Nutrition is a science
  - o Basic, social, applied and health sciences provide scientific evidence for nutrition
  - o Basic
    - ☐ Chemistry
    - • Food
    - • Metabolic functions
    - • Growth and development
  - o Social
    - ☐ Talk about the people
    - ☐ Talk about the behavior
    - ☐ Political (state and federal agencies)
    - • Where Federal regulations come from social science
    - • Laws and programs
    - • Research funding
    - • Public education
    - • Licensing
  - o Applied
    - ☐ Agriculture
    - ☐ Family and Consumer Science
  - o Health

- ☐ Chronic illnesses
- ☐ Disease prevention and control from nutrition
- • CDL Regulations
- o Division of Regulated Child Care (gov.)
- ☐ Sets minimum
- o STARS- voluntary agency for regulated child care (gov.)
- ☐ Goes a step past min.
- o National Assoc. for the Education of Young Children (Professional, NAEYC)
- ☐ Goes past the STARS, and gives national ranking
- o State and Federal for food
- ☐ Health Dept.
- • Inspection of Food prep
- • Kitchen safety and sanity
- ☐ USDA
- • Food program
- • Leading health problems
- o Diet related problems
- ☐ Heart diseases
- • Leading cause of death in America
- ☐ Cancers

- ☐ Diabetes mellitus
  - • Type I
  - • Type II
- ☐ Cirrhosis of the liver
  - • Alcohol (ETOH)
  - • Drug abuses
- ☐ Obesity
  - • 25% of the population is obese or overweight
- ☐ Malnutrition
- ☐ Eating disorder
  - • Anorexia Nervosa
  - • Bulimia
- ☐ Hypertension (high blood pressure)

However, there is more science in food than just nutritional science; there are multitudes of disciplines that play vital roles in our food system.

There is biology in food

Chemistry

- • Types of microorganisms that may lead to problems in our food supply?
  - • 4 types of food borne illnesses
  - o Bacteria
  - o Viruses

o   Parasites

o   Seafood

•   Specific federal agencies are charged by congress to protect public from food borne illnesses

•   HACCP

o   Is

•   HACCP's connection to the federal government and the public sector

•   Food additives

o   Do

o   Intentional

o   Incidental

•   5 types of additives

•   GRAS list

•   Delaney Clause

•   Process of approving food additive

•   Process of removing food additive

•   5 examples of "naturally occurring additives that may be harmful

•   Concerns about environmental contamination of food supply and system

•   Preventive ways to reduce risks in food supply

•   Trade-offs for consumers and families

- Things that are being done to address issues in food systems

- Laws that are working to address issues in food systems

- Preventable practices in food safety

-

- FDA
o Overseeing and protecting health, proper labeling
o Resources to the public
  □ Safety
  □ Guides
  □ Procedures
  □ Recalls
  □ Illnesses
o Oversees over one million organizations to promote good health and reduce food borne illness
o Maternal and child
  □ Red book
  • Toxicity
  • Fetus health
  • Vaccines
  • Obesity
  □ Substance abuse
o Enforcement

o   Health

o   Safety

o   Charged with public health safety for food and non-food products

o   Growth dev

☐   Prevent chronic diseases

☐   Managing Allergies in schools/child care

•   4-6%

☐   Reactions mostly happen at school

•   EPA

•   Environmental protection agency

o   Pesticides

o   Environment

o   Organics

o   Food illnesses

☐   3 billion annually

☐   900 deaths annually

☐   6.5-33 million annually

o   Asthma

o   Educational materials

☐   Consumer information

•   Monsanto

o   1901

o   Ag products

o   Volunteer

☐   20 volunteer hours =money

- ☐ Volunteer at food banks
- ☐ Donations, and the match the funds
- o Empowering farmers to produce more with less
- o Reducing on farm cost
- o GMO
- o Education
- ☐ Graduate grants
- ☐ Solve food insecurity issues
- o Consequences
- ☐ GMO wheat 2008
- • Contaminated
- • Economy crash
- • Asia pulled out from wheat purchases from the US
- o Biotechnology of food
- o GM seeds
- • Save the Children
- o Emergency
- o Distributing food, sanitation and hygiene
- ☐ Hurricanes, disasters, floods, storms, diseases outbreaks
- o Newborn, pregnant, infant health
- o To reduce the number of newborn deaths
- o Non-profit
- o Birth
- ☐ Colostrum at birth through breast milk
- o Established

- ☐ UK in 1919
- o Nutrition
- ☐ 1 million babies die per day
- ☐ 2 million die within a month
- ☐ Malnutrition= 3.1 mil child death
- ☐ 170 mil children fail to reach nutritional potential
- ☐ 2 bill suffer from nutrition decency
- ☐ Well-nourished
- • Economically secure
- • Do better in school
- • Contribute
- • Service learning
- o Civic engagement
- o Advocacy
- o Activism
- o Informing policy makers with
- ☐ Facts
- ☐ Figures
- ☐ Factors
- • CSA
- o Community supported agriculture
- o Description based farm
- ☐ Raise animals with
- • No GMO
- • No antibiotics
- • Sustainability

- ☐ Why
- • Buy local
- • Support local economy
- • Support sustainability
- • Fresh
- • 350 for a half stalk
- • Buy the share, get the crop
- ☐ For Pete's sake farm
- ☐ CSA Farmers
- • 35-45
- • Gender split at 50/50
- • 77% of CSA farmers are college graduates and 25% possess graduate degrees
- • Bill Best farm
- o Sustainable mountain agriculture center
- • Farm-to-School
- o complementary education
- o School farming
- o Regional food to schools
- o School gardening
- o Stats
- ☐ 40,000 schools, 40%+ of all US schools
- ☐ 26 states support this program
- ☐ National farm to school month- OCT
- o Research

☐   How to promote sustainable and healthy methods to children

o   Chef Ann Foundation

o   The LunchBox

o   The national school garden network

o   Gives the school

☐   Menu planning

☐   Defining and finding local foods

☐   Local food kit

•   CACFP

o   Child and Adult Care Food Program

•   Eight Reliable websites

o   DHHS

☐   Early detention and intervention

☐   Head start and intervention

o   USDA

☐   MyPlate

o   DEPT OF COMMERERCE-CENSUS DATA

o   CDC-VITAL STATS

o   NAEYC

☐   High quality research for early childhood

☐   For education and caretakers

☐   Transparency

☐   Reflection

☐   Collaboration

☐   Goals

- High quality early learning
- Education profession
- Organizational advancement
- Organizational excellence
- Leadership and innovation
- ☐ Vision
- All young children thrive and learn to reach their full potential
- This is accomplished through their organizational certification and accreditation
- Educational information for educators, caretakers, and parents
- ☐ Child nutrition
- CACFP
- o Two meals and one snack
- Special milk program
- National school lunch schools
- After school snacks
- o Operates and locates where 50% or more students can get free gov't foods
- ☐ Resources
- Conferences for professional
- Week of the young child
- Teacher and family activities
- For families
- o Picky eater
- o Ask a question

o   Blog

o   Help find childcare

o   AND

o   AA OF PEDS

☐   Membership based

☐   Resources for many age groups

☐   professionals

•   MDs

•   Surgeons

•   Nurses

•   Peds

☐   Sustains community based programs

☐   Education

•   Dept. of AAP education

o   Division of cont. med Edu

o   Workforce Edu policy

o   Life stupor

o   Human resources

o   Scholarly journal

o   IT

☐   Research

☐   Professional resources

•   Practice transformations

•   Clinical support

•   Journals and publications

•   Webinars

- Conferences
- Federal community and state nutrition program
- AAP oversees the congressional program to improve school lunch
  - Healthy hunger free act of 2010
- WIC
- School lunch
- School breakfast
  - Center for science for the public interest
  - NATL COUNCIL AGAINST HEALTH FRAUD- NCAHF
- Dr. Stephen Barrett, PHD, MD
- Health information
- Principles of science to enable consumers to make a conscious choice
- Accountability for law makers
- Principle
  - Everyone has a stake for high standards
  - Everyone shares responsibility
  - The scientific process is essential for proving safe
  - Accurately labeled
  - Consumer bills rights
- Education
-
  - Other Professional organizations
- American cancer society

- ☐ Amer heart, diabetes, dental, associations
- ☐ Natl cancer institute
- • CDL
- o Go as a team
- o Written plan
- ☐ Submit deadline
- • GOOD FRIDAY
- • April 3rd
- ☐ Outlines
- • Objectives
- o Developmentally appropriate for age
- o Tammy Carter (as. Dir.) email for concerns
- • Date and Time
- o Within guidelines for when the project will take place
- o Complete my the 24th of April
- o Reflection
- ☐ Larger issues discussed in class
- • Infant morality
- • GMO/ Monsanto
- • Civic engagement
- •

- • Digestion absorption and utilization
- o Portion size
- o Peanuts

- ☐ Legumes
- • Beans
- • Protein
- o Nitrogen
- ☐ Provides growth for soil plants
- ☐ That why protein promotes growth and development
- • CHO
- o Starch
- o Fiber
- o Candy
- ☐ CHO
- • Sugar
- o Pizza
- ☐ Topping
- • Cheese
- o Protein
- o Calcium
- o Vit
- ☐ A, D, B
- o Fat
- o Zinc
- o Potassium
- • Meat
- o Protein
- o fat

- Sauce
o Tomato
o Antioxidants
☐ Dough
- Grains
o Digestion
☐ Breaks down food so that it can be absorbed and fiber can help move waste
☐ Essential so the body can use the food
☐ Cannot occur without PRO
☐ Nutrients cant preform with the food being broken down
- Nutrients that need to be broken down
o CHO (at least 40% of cal. should be CHO to prevent ketosis)
o Ketosis (dangerous for low or no CHO diet) high levels of ketones in the blood, which shuts off EMZ functions where organs can't function
o When the kidney tries to excrete ketones, the kidney removes electrolytes
o For diabetics, ketosis can kill them in a matter of hours
☐ Monosaccharides
- Glucose
- Fructose
- Mannose
- Galactose

- FAT
  - Fatty Acids
    - Hydrophobic
  - Glycerol
    - Water soluble alcohol
    - Hydrophilic
- PRO
  - Amino acids
    - EAA
    - NEAA

- Suffixes
- –ase = enzyme
- –saccharide= CHO
- –ose= sugar
  - Disaccharides
- Formulas
  - Glucose + Galactose= Lactose
  - Glucose + Fructose= Sucrose
  - Glucose + Glucose= Maltose
- Types
  - Lactose
    - Enzyme Lactase breaks down Lactose
    - This break down is caused by PRO
    - Breaks down to

o   Glucose + Galactose

•   If the Lactose is not broken down (Lactose intolerance) the bacteria in the colon will ferment the lactose and

☐   Sucrose (less than 10% of CHO should be sucrose)

•   EMZ sucrose

•   Breaks down to

o   Glucose + Fructose

•   Sugar added

o   Sucrose added

•   No sugar added

o   Sugar present, but no sucrose

☐   maltose

•   EMZ maltase

•   Breaks down to

o   Glucose + Glucose

•   Glucose is the preferred source of energy for brain cells

•   Aerobic produces ATP (stored energy)

II.

Book of Exercise:

Why Food is Not Enough

"People who want to live, actually live. They do not sit all day, watch television or lay around. People that want to live are active"

-Getting Started-

I remember stepping onto my college campus on the first day of orientation week filled with excitement and anticipation. I was eleven hours away from home, and finally on my own. It was at this moment, that for the first time I was making all of the decisions.

III.

Book of Water and Digestion:

A Detailed Look at Water and the Gastrointestinal Tract

"Think about it, how long would your car run without gasoline, how stiff would it be without oil, or how hard would it be hard would driving be without fluids.

Now think of your body."

-Getting Started-

I remember stepping onto my college campus on the first day of orientation week filled with excitement and anticipation. I was eleven hours away from home, and finally on my own. It was at this moment, that for the first time I was making all of the decisions.

IV.

Book of Lipids:

Understanding Good and Bad Fats

"""

-Getting Started-

I remember stepping onto my college campus on the first day of orientation week filled with excitement and anticipation. I was eleven hours away from home, and finally on my own. It was at this moment, that for the first time I was making all of the decisions.

V.

Book of Protein:

The Science and Sources of Protein

"Strength is deeper than physical strength. Being strong is not just how many weights you can pick up, but being strong is how many poor habits you can put down"

-Getting Started-

I remember stepping onto my college campus on the first day of orientation week filled with excitement and anticipation. I was eleven hours away from home, and finally on my own. It was at this moment, that for the first time I was making all of the decisions.

VI.

Book of Vitamins and Minerals:

Understanding the Purpose and Functions of Vitamins and Minerals

"If vitamins are in real food, then we shouldn't need vitamin supplements unless our food isn't..."

-Getting Started-

I remember stepping onto my college campus on the first day of orientation week filled with excitement and anticipation. I was eleven hours away from home, and finally on my own. It was at this moment, that for the first time I was making all of the decisions.

VII.

Book of Carbohydrates :

How Carbs are Hidden and Affect Everyone's Diet

"It is surprising that so many people count the amount of sugar they consume but have no idea what carbs are. There is a scary science to carbs- they react in the body similarly to candy, soda or anything else with sugar"

-Getting Started-

I remember stepping onto my college campus on the first day of orientation week filled with excitement and anticipation. I was eleven hours away from home, and finally on my own. It was at this moment, that for the first time I was making all of the decisions.

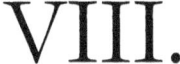

Book of Sugar:

How Sugar Affects the Body

*"My grandmother's generation called diabetes, 'sugar'.
That's interesting, that we never got the connection"*

-Getting Started-

I remember stepping onto my college campus on the first
day of orientation week filled with excitement and
anticipation. I was eleven hours away from home, and
finally on my own. It was at this moment, that for the first
time I was making all of the decisions.

IX.

Book of Budget:

How I Became Interested in Nutrition

"There is an epidemic where people who are working, still cannot afford to eat. We are living in a food famine, the reason that we don't know this, is because we are surrounded by food"

-Getting Started-

I remember stepping onto my college campus on the first day of orientation week filled with excitement and anticipation. I was eleven hours away from home, and finally on my own. It was at this moment, that for the first time I was making all of the decisions.

X.

Book of Labels and Deceptions:

How to Understand Food Labels

"Riddle: Who am I?

I told a man he was buying food. I sold him plastic.

Answer: Food Companies"

-Getting Started-

I remember stepping onto my college campus on the first day of orientation week filled with excitement and anticipation. I was eleven hours away from home, and finally on my own. It was at this moment, that for the first time I was making all of the decisions.

XII.

Book of DOH:

Diabetes. Obesity. Heart Disease.

"If you think that health problems can be solved by curing obesity, you are very wrong. First you must answer why obesity is a problem that needs curing"

-Getting Started-

I remember stepping onto my college campus on the first day of orientation week filled with excitement and anticipation. I was eleven hours away from home, and finally on my own. It was at this moment, that for the first time I was making all of the decisions.

XII.

Book of Getting Started:

How I Became Interested in Nutrition

"The importance of a goal should not first be in setting a date to accomplish that goal, but the first step should be determining when you are truly ready to begin"

-Getting Started-

I remember stepping onto my college campus on the first day of orientation week filled with excitement and anticipation. I was eleven hours away from home, and finally on my own. It was at this moment, that for the first time I was making all of the decisions.

Afterword

Now that you have this knowledge, it is totally up to you to make any change that you think are necessary. But remember the changes that you make today, will always affect your tomorrows, regardless of whether those changes were good or bad. To all of you who wanted information, I have given you SOME in this book. This is not a one-stop train in the pursuit of nutrition; the goal was for this to be the first stop on the tracks to wellness. I hope that this has given you some insight to food, but I hope further, that it ignited a fire inside of you, one that burns calories but also drives you to learn more. We are all students in this pursuit of knowledge and healthier lives; let our journeys continue.

www.ingramcontent.com/pod-product-compliance
Lightning Source LLC
Chambersburg PA
CBHW020402290526
45785CB00005B/2412